Dr Pauline Hili completed a degree in Chemistry & Biochemistry in Melbourne, Australia. She undertook a PhD at the University of Westminster examining the antimicrobial activity of essential oils and looking into their mode of action. Pauline is Technical Director for the world renowned Neal's Yard Remedies and has gained a wealth of experience formulating aromatherapy based products, some of which is shared here.

Pauline has lectured on essential oils internationally, and she also teaches on Neal's Yard Remedies' course in Aromatherapy and Essential Oil Science.

THE ANTIMICROBIAL PROPERTIES OF ESSENTIAL OILS

DR PAULINE HILI

Winter Press
16 Stambourne Way
West Wickham
Kent BR4 9NF

First published by Winter Press in 2001

ISBN 1 874581 83 5

Cover design by Rachel Codd at Neal's Yard Remedies

Printed by Biddles of Guildford, Surrey

This book is presented as a collection of scientific results and recipes. It is not intended to replace or supersede professional consultation or treatment and no guarantee can be given as to the efficacy or appropriateness of a remedy in an individual case without professional advice.

ACKNOWLEDGEMENTS

This book is the fruit of a collaboration between my employer, Neal's Yard Remedies, and the Department of Biological Science at the University of Westminster.

I would like to extend my grateful thanks to Romy Fraser of Neal's Yard Remedies and to my Professor at the University of Westminster, Christine Evans. These two people created the context for the whole thing to happen.

Thanks also to all my colleagues at Neal's Yard Remedies. And to Susan Curtis and Colin Winter of Winter Press for their faith in turning this into a book and their patient editing.

Contents

Preface

We live in a scientific world as evidenced by cars, aeroplanes, computers, mobile phones, pre-prepared meals and health care products - for which we demand high standards of reliability, safety and fitness for purpose. Such demands impose rigorous testing to ensure quality products. Science must meet these demands, while the public has a right to demand quality in all commercial products.

Products that have a proven use over many centuries include plant essential oils. They have been used widely since the 6th century BC, when no scientific testing, how we understand it today, was performed. Their use has continued into the 21st century because they are 'known to work'. But today's public demands greater product safety than ever before, so the effects of essential oils must be scientifically proven to guarantee reliability, safety and efficacy.

This manual links the traditional uses of essential oils with rigorous scientific examination of their potency as preservatives and anti-microbial agents. With this detailed knowledge we can begin to appreciate and understand why our ancestors found them to be effective remedies for a wide range of symptoms. Understanding the specific properties of each essential oil has led to the customised design of products for individual ailments. Some of these products are described here.

Professor Christine Evans
University of Westminster
London, 2001

Introduction

The Antimicrobial History of Essential Oils

Essential oils have been used for their antimicrobial properties since ancient times. The oldest still for producing essential oils that has been found is from the Indus Valley of what is now Pakistan, and is 5,000 years old. The Egyptians are known to have used essential oils for embalming and to help preserve the flesh from microbial decay. The Greeks continued the use of oils, and used them both medicinally and cosmetically. The Romans who popularised the concept of bathing, used aromatic oils for massaging and purifying the skin. One of the earliest records of the use of essential oils is for the oil of turpentine. The Roman historian Pliny (484-425 BC), and his contemporary Dioscorides, mention oil of turpentine and give partial information about the method of producing it.

Following the spread of knowledge on aromatic oils and perfumes via the crusades to the Far East and Arabia, it is believed the Arabic physician named Avicenna rediscovered the process of distillation. Initially distillation was used primarily for the production of scented water with the oil that crystallized out, being considered an undesirable by-product.

A Catalan physician of the 13th century, Arnald de Villanova, is believed to be one of the first doctors to have used essential oils as we know them today, and prescribed them for their therapeutic value. Arnald de Villanova's praise of the remedial qualities of distilled waters and oils resulted in the process of distillation becoming a speciality in medieval and post-medieval pharmacies.

In the second half of the 16th century Reiff (1556) published his book in which he referred to clove, mace, nutmeg, anise, spice and cinnamon for their therapeutic value.

By the 17th century the preserving qualities of essential oils were well known and used by the pharmacists of the day. Quercetanus (1544- 1609) in his famous "Pharmcopoeia Dogmaticorum Restituta" praised the use of small quantities of essential oils applied directly for their healing properties.

In the 19th century considerable research was conducted on the nature of essential oils and aromatic compounds. Physical and chemical procedures were established for the analysis of aromatics. Standards were prepared for wide-spread use and referencing.

In the early 20th century the discovery of the relationship which exists between microorganisms and disease brought forth a more extensive use of essential oils and their isolates for the purpose of controlling microbial growth. Some of the earliest physicians and scientists to have written on the antimicrobial activity of essential oils include Schonbein (1840), Miller (1892), Harlan (1888) and Mawhinney (1900).

One of the earliest recorded scientific investigations into the antiseptic powers of essential oils was in 1887 by Chamberlain. Using the Koch thread method and suspending bacteria in sealed tubes over the respective oils, Chamberlain found that with cinnamon oil 4 days was required to kill anthrax spores, whereas the vegetative cells were killed in 65 hours. He also found origanum, angelica and geranium oils to have activity against the vegetative spores.

Rene Maurice Gattefossé first coined the term aromatherapie in a scientific paper on the healing properties of essential oils which was published in 1928. Other French doctors have continued with this work. Jean Valnet a former army surgeon used essential oils to treat severe burns and battle injuries, and went on to publish the classic text book "The Practice of Aromatherapy".

Martindale (1910) published the results of the first extensive research on the bactericidal properties of essential oils using quantitative test procedures. Using both aqueous and soap solutions of oils and comparing activity of the oils to phenol, Martindale tested more than 50 different oils and their isolates using *Escherichia coli* as the test organism. Among the most active were cinnamon, clove and thyme oil.

Cavel (1918) conducted extensive research on the antimicrobial properties of oils on a number of sewage microrganisms. His data showed thyme, oreganum, cassia, rose and clove were most potent at inhibiting the growth of microorganisms found in sewage.

Starting in 1956, Maruzzella and co-workers published some 18 papers on the antimicrobial properties of essential oils and aromatic perfumery chemicals.

During the 1970 – 1980's a large number of studies on the antimicrobial activity of essential oils have been performed. It became recognised that testing and evaluation of essential oils was difficult because of their volatility, their water insolubility and their complexity. Comparisons between laboratories was very difficult because of the wide variation in techniques and lack of information on the composition of oils.

Modern studies are presented with detailed information regarding the chemical composition of essential oils and paying particular attention to the strain number of the test organisms.

Some new and exciting research into essential oils has been conducted in recent years.

The Department of Physiology and Pharmacology, University of Ceara, Brazil; has recently published a paper showing the anti-inflammmatory and antinoceptive effects of 1,8-cineole terpenoid oxide present in many essential oils such as cinnamon and clove. (Phytotherapy Research, 2000 June, 14 (4):240-4)

Satureja hortensis L. (Lamiaceae) is an annual herb that is used traditionally in Iran for treating stomach and intestinal disorders. Recent work has shown that it displays antispasmodic activity in vitro and the essential oil of this plant at low doses inhibited castor oil induced diarrhoea in mice. It was concluded that the oil may have some clinical benefit in the treatment of such gastrointestinal disorders such as colic and further work should be conducted. (Journal Ethnopharmacology, 2000 July; 71 (1-2): 187-92)

The use of aromatherapy in midwifery practice has been examined with a recent study investigating the contribution of aromatherapy to the promotion of maternal comfort during labor and as a tool to aid and improve the quality of midwifery care. A total of 8,058 mothers where evaluated and the women where offered aromatherapy to relieve anxiety, pain, nausea or to strengthen contractions. The results showed that the use of aromatherapy during childbirth was an increasingly popular care option for both mothers and midwives. More than 50% of the mothers rated it as helpful. (Journal Alternative and Complementary Medicine, 2000 April, 6 (2):141-7)

The psychological effects of aromatherapy on 14 female patients who were being treated for chronic hemodialysis was recently investigated. The results showed that in chronic hemodialysis patients aromatherapy using hiba oil provided an effective, non-invasive means for the treatment of depression and anxiety, and that lavender alleviated the anxiety. (Psychiatry Clinical Neuroscience, 2000 August; 54 (4), 393-7)

A recent study has examined by GC-MS analysis some essential oils from some Greek aromatic plants and looked at their fungitoxicity against *Penicillium digitatum*. (J. Agric. Food Chem. 2000 June; 48(6): 2576-81)

A regular look at the scientific journals will show how work in the field of essential oil chemistry and aromatherapy is continuing to grow. The field is alive with possibilities to provide alternatives to some of our modern drugs, pesticides and chemicals. Plants can provide a renewable non polluting solution to a number of our modern day problems. Further research is required to continue to uncover the value of phytochemicals in our modern lives.

Chapter 1

The Biological and Ecological Roles of Essential Oils in the Plant

Many theories have arisen as to the biological and ecological roles of essential oils.

In the past it was thought that essential oils were waste products or storage compounds.

It is only in recent times that we have began to uncover a wealth of information on the biological and ecological roles of essential oils. The function of essential oils is believed to be largely communicative, and a variety of complex interactions have evolved enabling plants to utilise essential oils to influence their environment. Research has shown volatile oils to be active in the attraction of pollinators e.g. insects; as dispersal agents; in plant-plant interactions; as defencc compounds against insects and animals; and as antifungal and antibacterial agents.

An example of essential oils performing a communication role in plant-plant interactions can be found with the bitter orange tree (*Citrus aurantium*) and its relationship with a pigweed (*Amaranthus retroflexus*) which can be found growing in its vicinity. The bitter orange tree produces an oil containing high amounts of alpha and beta pinene, limonene and citronellal which are known to cause inhibition in the growth and development of the pigweed. (Al Saadawi et al, 1985).

Plant interactions with insects and animals may also be mediated through essential oils. The presence of an essential oil containing high levels of linalool in the peel of citrus fruit confers resistance to attack by the Caribbean fruit fly (*Anastrepha suspensa*) (Greany et al, 1983).

The volatile monoterpenes that comprise about half of the oleoresin produced by certain species of conifer act as phytoprotective agents, defending the tree from herbivore and pathogen attack (Gijzen et al, 1991).

The delineation of their protected territory by marking grass stems with droplets of a fluid secreted from their enlarged mandibular glands by *Centris adani*, provides an example of the role of essential oils in the defence mechanisms of insects. The odiferous fluid contains geraniol, nerol, neral and geranyl acetate (Vinson et al 1982).

Essential oils isolated from leaves and seeds of seven umbelliferous plants have recently been tested against the growth of mould *Aspergillus flavus* (Dwivedi and Dubey, 1993). Those from the seeds of *Trachyspermum ammi, Cuminum cyminum, Carum carvi, Daucus carota* and the leaves of *Anethum graveolens* exhibited antifungal activity against the test organism. Amongst these, oil from seeds of *Trachyspermum ammi* was most toxic. The fungitoxicity potency of *Trachyspermum* seed oil remained unchanged after a long storage period and at high inoculum density of the test fungus. The oil was thermostable and was more efficacious than some commercially available fungicides.

Essential oils also act as antifeedants, with components of oils of shrubs and conifers inhibiting rumen microorganisms upon which ruminants rely for digestion of plant material (van Beck and de Groot, 1986).

The Effects of Essential Oils on Microorganisms

The antimicrobial activity of essential oils has been well documented, but very little is known about the precise mechanism by which this effect is exerted.

A study in the 1980s examined the effects of geraniol, a common component in the essential oils of geranium and palmarosa, on the membrane function of strains of *Candida* and *Saccharomyces* (Bard et al 1988).

Geraniol inhibits the growth of *Candida albicans* and *Saccharomyces cerevisiae*. It was shown to enhance the rate of potassium leakage out of whole cells and also shown by fluorescence polarisation to increase membrane fluidity of *C. albicans*. Biophysical studies using differential scanning calorimetry, fluorescence polarisation and osmotic swelling of phospholipid vesicles demonstrated that geraniol decreased the phase-transition temperature of dipalmitoylphosphatidylcholine vesicles, affected fluidity throughout the bilayer and caused an increase in bilayer permeability to erythritol.

The action of terpenoids on energy metabolism in the bacterium *Rhodopseudomonas sphaeroides* (ATCC 17023) has been examined (Knobloch et al 1986). Twenty-five different terpenoic compounds were tested. Most of the essential oil components tested inhibited both respiratory electron flow and coupled oxidative phosphorylation. Among the components tested, thymol, carvarol and other alcohols were the most potent inhibitors, influencing electron flow and ATP synthesis even at a concentration of 0.02mM.

The interaction of cyclic hydrocarbons with biological membranes has been studied (Sikkema et al 1994). The membrane-buffer partition coefficient of these cyclic hydrocarbons revealed that these compounds preferentially reside in the membrane. The partition coefficients closely correlated with the partition coefficients of the same compounds in a standard octanol-water system. The accumulation of hydrocarbon molecules resulted in swelling of the membrane bilayer. Parallel to the expansion of the membrane, an increase in the membrane fluidity was observed. These effects on the integrity of the membrane caused an increased passive flux of protons and carboxyfluorescein.

In proteoliposomes containing cytochrome c oxidase both components of the proton motive force, the pH gradient and the electrical potential were dissipated with increasing concentrations of cyclic hydrocarbons. At higher concentrations, cytochrome c oxidase was also inactivated. The effective concentrations of the different cyclic hydrocarbons correlated with their partition coefficients between the membrane and aqueous phase. It was concluded that the impairment of microbial activity by the cyclic hydrocarbons most likely resulted from hydrophobic interaction with the membrane, which affects the functioning of the membrane and membrane-embedded proteins.

The action of eucalyptol on *Candida albicans* has been studied using transmission and scanning electronmicroscopy (Steinmetz et al 1988). Yeast cells exposed for three hours to eucalyptol dissolved in Tween 80 appeared distorted and atypical aspects of cell division were observed. Membranous rolls and polysaccharide heaps were noted in the cytoplasm. Following exposure for five hours the yeast cells were degraded and perforated and their cytoplasmic contents were released through the perforations. The cell walls of dead yeasts seemed intact and hence the cells showed no modification in the exterior aspects. Following treatment for twenty-four hours, observations showed only a little plaiting and no perforation. The fungicidal action was not increased in spite of the longer contact time.

The Antimicrobial Activity of Essential Oils

The use of essential oils as antimicrobial agents has been described for many years, starting with the phenol coefficients of a number of essential oils published by Martindale in 1910. Some more modern examples of in vitro testing of the antimicrobial activity of essential oils follows. There are also some direct links to be drawn between some specific pathogens and certain clinical diseases.

In 1992 the antifungal activity of six essential oils were tested in vitro against sixteen clinical isolates of the dermatophytes *Epidermophyton floccosum, Microsporum canis, Trichophyton mentagrophytes* and *Trichophyton rubrum* isolated from patients with dermatophytosis (Lima et al). The oils were obtained from the plants *Annona classiflora*, cinnamon (*Cinnamomum zeylanicum*), lemongrass (*Cymbopogon citratus*), East Indian basil (*Ocimum gratissimum*), *Proium heptaphyllum* and *Xylopin frutesens.* Oils (with the exception of that from *P. heptaphyllem*) caused inhibition of 81% of the studied strains of dermatophytes. Only two strains of *Trichophyton rubrum* and one of *Microsporum canis* were resistant.

The production of Aflatoxin B1 by *Aspergillus flavus* in the presence of cinnamon, clove and cardamom oils has been studied. Growth and aflatoxin B1 production was inhibited by 0.5 $\mu l\ ml^{-1}$ cinnamon oil and by 1 $\mu l\ ml^{-1}$ clove oil (Patkar et al 1993).

The development of resistance of periodontal pathogens to antibiotics has become a major concern among dental practitioners. The use of plant derived antimicrobial agents are being investigated. The essential oils of *Foeniculum vulgare* (wild fennel seed) and *Syzygium aromaticum* (clove) have been tested and demonstrate promising results for their antimicrobial activity against oral pathogenic bacteria.

Both oils inhibited the growth of *Streptococcus sanguis, S. salivarius, S. gordonii, Porphyromonas gingivatis* and *Prevotella intermedia* with an inhibition zone diameter on agar plates ranging from 8mm to 47mm (Branchmays et al, 1994).

Many AIDS patients develop fungal infections. Yeast like some *Candida* species and mainly *Cryptococcus neoformans* appear in the last period of the illness often resulting in death of the patient. In 1992, *Cryptococcus neoformans* was diagnosed among 4 % of patients with AIDS in Europe, 12 % in the USA and 33 % in East Africa.

It has been shown that *Cryptococcus neoformans* is inhibited in vitro by *Cymbopogon martinii* (palmarosa), or *Cinnamomum zeylanicum* (cinnamon) oils. The minimum inhibitory concentration (MIC) of palmarosa oil was 200 μl L^{-1} and the minimum fungicidal concentration (MFC) was 200 mcg L(-1). The MIC of cinnamon oil was 100 μl L^{-1} and the MFC was 250 μl L^{-1} (Viollon and Chaumont, 1994).

Food borne illness resulting from the consumption of food contaminated with pathogenic bacteria and/or their toxins is of vital concern to public health. Of food borne outbreaks in the USA during 1983-1987, 66 % were caused by bacterial pathogens (Bean et al, 1990).

On the 14th January 1997 it was reported that since 22nd November 1996, sixteen people had died in Wishaw, Scotland, from *Eschericha coli* 0157 food poisoning, making this one of the most serious outbreaks of *E. coli* food poisoning ever. Over four hundred people were affected. In 1996, 9,500 people in Japan were affected by an outbreak of *E. coli 0157* food poisoning and eleven people died.

Antibacterial activity of eleven essential oil components against five food borne pathogens, *E. coli, E. coli 0157:H7, Salmonella typhimurium, Listeria monocytogenes* and *Vibrio vulnificus* has been tested (Kim et al, 1995). Carvacrol showed strong bactericidal activity against all tester strains, while limonene, nerolidol, and beta-ionone were mostly inactive. Carvacrol was highly bactericidal against *S. typhimurium* and *V. vulnificus* in liquid medium with a Minimum Bactericidal Concentration (MBC) of 250 $\mu l\ ml^{-1}$. Citral and perillaldehyde had MBCs of 100 and 250 $\mu l\ ml^{-1}$ against *V. vulnificus*. Terpineol and linalool were least potent, with MBCs of 1000 $\mu l\ ml^{-1}$. Citral, geraniol and perillaldehyde at 500$\mu l\ ml^{-1}$ completely killed *E. coli, E. coli 0157:H7* and *S. typhimurium*, while citronellal at 250 $\mu l\ ml^{-1}$ killed *V. vulnificus*.

Many of these compounds are classified as "Generally Recognised As Safe" (GRAS) in European pharmaceutical classifications and therefore could serve as potential antibacterial agents to inhibit pathogen growth in food.

The following chart has been compiled from a large number of research programmes carried out world wide during the 1990s. The essential oils listed have all been shown to be very active against the microorganisms shown in vitro (for references see Appendix). The diseases associated with the microorganisms are also listed, but the appropriate clinical application of the essential oils is down to the art of the aromatherapist!

SOME COMMON MICROORGANISMS, ASSOCIATED CONDITIONS AND ACTIVE ESSENTIAL OILS

MICROORGANISM	CONDITION	REPUTED OILS*
Bacillus cereus	Food poisoning	Basil Cinnamon Clove Rosemary
Bordetella pertussis	Whooping cough	Basil Cypress Rosemary Thyme
Candida albicans	Thrush	Palmarosa Sage
Cornybacterium *Propionibacterium* *Streptococcus*	Body odour	Cinnamon Clove Coriander Lemongrass
Diplococcus pneumoniae	Conjunctivitis	Chamomile, Blue Lemon Lemongrass
Escherichia coli	Cystitis Enteritis Pyelitis	Clove Coriander Palmarosa Peppermint Thyme
Leptotrichia buccalis *Streptococcus mutans*	Plaque	Cinnamon
Pityrosporum ovale *Pityrosporum orbicular*	Dandruff	Rosemary Cedarwood
Propionibacteria (formerly *Corynebacteria*)	Acne	Cajeput Lavender Juniper

MICROORGANISM	CONDITION	REPUTED OILS*
Pseudomonas aerugenosa	Eye infections	Chamomile Palmarosa Lemon
Salmonella enteritis	Food poisoning	Thyme Peppermint Coriander
Staphylococcus aureus	Boils Styes Conjunctivitis	Chamomile Clove Thyme Lemon
Streptococcus mutans	Tooth decay Halitosis	Nutmeg Peppermint Rosemary Clove Sage Myrrh
Streptococcus pyogens	Tonsillitis	Geranium Ginger Lemon Thyme Sage
Trichophyton mentagophytes	Athlete's Foot	Palmarosa Thyme Garlic Lemon Ho
Trichophyton violaceum	Ringworm	Garlic Tea tree

*See Appendix for list of References

Chapter 2

Activity of Essential Oils Against Microorganisms

WHICH OILS FOR WHICH MICROORGANISMS?

In my own study to establish which essential oils were most active against which bacteria and fungi, 50 different varieties of essential oil were investigated for their effects on 7 microorganisms.

The following microorganisms were used for these studies in plate testings (Hili et al 1997):

3 Bacteria
Escherichia coli NCTC 10418
Staphylococcus aureus NCTC 6571
Pseudomonas aerugenosa NCTC 10662

4 Yeasts
Candida albicans NCPF 113
Schizosaccharomyces pombe CMI 124
Saccharomyces cerevisiae CMI 61302
Torulopis utilus CMI 23311

The table overleaf summarises the results.

ESSENTIAL OILS TESTED

Oil	Species	Family	Part	Method	Bacteria: E. coli	Bacteria: S. aureus	Bacteria: P. aerugenosa	Yeasts: C. albicans	Yeasts: S. pombe	Yeasts: S. cerevisiae	Yeasts: T. utilus
Anise, Star	*Illicium verum*	Illiceaceae	Fruit	sd	1	0	0	1	2	1	2
Basil	*Ocimum basilicum*	Lamiaceae	Herb	sd	0	0	0	p	2	2	2
Bergamot	*Citrus bergamia*	Rutaceae	Rind	e	0	0	0	2	2	2	3
Black Pepper	*Piper nigrum*	Piperaceae	Fruit	sd	0	0	0	1	2	2	2
Cajuput	*Melaleuca cajiputi*	Myrtaceae	Twig/leaf	sd	1	0	0	2	p	2	2
Cardamom	*Elettaria cardamomum*	Zingiberaceae	Fruit	sd	1	1	0	1	p	2	2
Cedarwood	*Cedrus atlantica*	Pinaceae	Wood	sd	1	0	0	1	1	0	1
Chamomile, Blue	*Matricaria chamomilla*	Asteraceae	Flowers	sd	0	0	0	p	p	2	2
Chamomile, Roman	*Anthemis nobilis*	Asteraceae	Flowers	sd	0	0	0	2	2	2	2
Cinnamon	*Cinnamomum zeylanicum*	Lauraceae	Leaf	sd	3	3	2	2	3	3	3
Clary Sage	*Salvia sclarea*	Lamiaceae	Herb	sd	0	0	0	0	1	1	1
Clove	*Eugenia caryophyllata*	Myrtaceae	Leaf	sd	2	2	2	3	2	3	2
Coriander	*Coriandrum sativum*	Umbelliferae	Fruit	sd	2	2	1	2	2	2	2
Cypress	*Cupressus sempervirens*	Cupressaceae	Needles	sd	1	0	0	2	2	2	2
Eucalyptus, Blue Gum	*Eucalyptus globulus*	Myrtaceae	Leaves	sd	0	0	0	2	p	p	2
Eucalyptus citriodora	*Eucalyptus citriodora*	Myrtaceae	Leaves	sd	0	0	0	1	2	2	1
Fennel	*Foeniculum dulce*	Umbelliferae	Seeds	sd	0	0	0	1	2	2	2
Geranium	*Pelargonium graveolens*	Geraniaceae	Leaf/stem	sd	0	0	0	2	2	2	2
Ginger	*Zingiber officinalis*	Zingiberaceae	Root	sd	0	0	0	0	2	2	1
Grapefruit	*Citrus paradisi*	Rutaceae	Rind	e	0	0	0	1	2	2	2
Ho Leaf	*Cinnamomum camphora*	Lauraceae	Leaf	sd	2	2	1	2	3	3	2
Jasmine, Absolute	*Jasminum officinalis*	Oleaceae	Flowers	ab	0	0	0	0	p	0	0
Juniper	*Juniperus communis*	Cupressaceae	Twig/needle	sd	0	0	0	1	p	2	1
Juniperberry	*Juniperus communis*	Cupressaceae	Berries	sd	0	0	0	1	p	p	1
Lavender	*Lavandula angustifolia*	Lamiaceae	Flowers	sd	2	0	1	2	3	3	2
Lemon	*Citrus limonum*	Rutaceae	Rind	e	0	0	0	p	p	2	2
Lemongrass	*Cymbopogon citratus*	Gramineae	Herb	sd	p	p	p	p	p	p	2

					Bacteria			Yeasts			
Lime	*Citrus aurantifolia*	Rutaceae	Fruit	sd	0	0	0	2	2	2	2
Mandarin	*Citrus reticulata*	Rutaceae	Rind	e	0	0	0	1	2	2	1
Marjoram, Spanish	*Thymus mastichina*	Lamiaceae	Herb	sd	2	2	1	1	2	2	1
Melissa	*Melissa officinalis*	Lamiaceae	Herb	sd	0	0	0	2	2	2	2
Myrrh	*Commiphora molmol*	Burseraceae	Resin	sd	2	p	p	p	p	p	p
Neroli	*Citrus aurantium*	Rutaceae	Flowers	sd	1	2	0	2	2	2	1
Olibanum	*Boswellia thurifera*	Burseraceae	Resin	sd	0	0	0	1	2	2	1
Orange, Sweet	*Citrus sinensis*	Rutaceae	Rind	e	0	0	0	2	2	2	2
Palmarosa	*Cymbopogon martinii*	Gramineae	Herb	sd	0	2	1	2	2	2	2
Patchouli	*Pogostemon patchoulii*	Lamiaceae	Herb	sd	0	0	0	1	1	1	1
Peppermint	*Mentha piperita*	Lamiaceae	Herb	sd	2	2	1	2	2	2	2
Petitgrain	*Citrus aurantium*	Rutaceae	Leaf/twig	sd	0	0	0	2	2	2	2
Pine	*Pinus sylvestris*	Pinaceae	Needles	sd	0	0	0	1	1	2	2
Rose otto	*Rosa centafolia*	Rosaceae	Petals	sd	p	p	1	1	1	1	1
Rose absolute	*Rosa damascena*	Rosaceae	Petals	ab	0	0	0	1	1	1	1
Rosemary	*Rosmarinus officinalis*	Lamiaceae	Herb	sd	1	0	0	1	2	2	1
Sage	*Salvia officinalis*	Lamiaceae	Herb	sd	2	1	0	2	2	1	2
Sandalwood	*Santalum album*	Santalaceae	Wood	sd	0	0	0	1	1	1	1
Tagettes	*Tagetes erecta*	Asteraceeae	Floweres	sd	0	p	0	1	2	1	1
Tea Tree	*Melaleuca alternifolia*	Myrtaceae	Leaves	sd	2	1	1	2	2	2	3
Thyme	*Thymus vulgaris*	Lamiaceae	Herb	sd	3	3	2	3	3	3	3
Vetiver	*Vetivera zizanoides*	Gramineae	Herb	sd	0	0	0	1	2	2	1
Ylang Ylang	*Cananga odorata*	Anonaceae	Flowers	sd	0	0	0	0	0	0	0

Key to Extraction **Method**
sd=Steam distilled,
e=Expression,
ab=Absolute (solvent extraction)

Figures refer to zone of inhibition for a minimum of three replicates. Maximum plate diameter was 80mm:
0 = zero,
1 = low (1-10mm mean diameter),
2 = moderate (11-39mm mean diameter)
3 = high (40-80mm mean diameter)
p = patches of inhibition but no clear area

As can be seen from the table above, the oils inhibited the growth of the yeast species more than the bacterial species. This confirms previous work (eg Hammerschmidt et al, 1993). *Pseudomonas aerugenosa* proved to be the most resistant organism, with only 11 of the 50 oils showing any significant inhibitory activity. *Staphylococcus aureus* proved to be the second most resistant organism, with only 12 oils showing activity, and 18 oils showed activity against *Escherichia coli.*

Regarding the yeasts, 41 oils showed inhibitory activity against *Candida albicans*, 43 oils showed activity against *Saccharomyces cerevisiae* and 47 showed activity against *Torulopis utilis.*

The level of inhibitory activity varied from low to high, or more precisely from 0.3 % to 90 % of total plate area.

The citrus oils, which included bergamot, grapefruit, lemon, lime, mandarin and orange showed no inhibition against the 3 bacterial species, which correlates with previous work.

Essential oils from spice plants are known to have excellent antimicrobial properties. The essential oils of cinnamon, clove and coriander showed strong inhibition of growth against all 7 microorganisms. Both cinnamon and clove oils contain eugenol as a major component. Eugenol is a substituted phenol, possessing strong antimicrobial activity. It is also found in Spanish marjoram oil, which also showed strong activity against all 7 microorganisms.

Coriander oil does not contain any of the major components found in clove and cinnamon oils. The major components of coriander oil are linalool and alpha-pinene. Linalool has previously been reported to have good inhibitory properties against *Candida albicans, Escherichia coli* and *Staphylococcus aureus.* It is also a major component in Spanish marjoram (16 %), lavender (24 %) and ho leaf oils (44 %).

Spanish marjoram and ho leaf oils showed activity against all seven microorganisms. Lavender oil showed activity against all organisms except for *S. aureus* which would suggest the antimicrobial activity of Spanish marjoram and ho leaf oils are not solely due to their linalool content.

Comparison of the activity of *Eucalyptus globulus* oil, which contains high amounts of 1-8 cineole, to *Eucalyptus citriodora* oil, which contains high amounts of citronellal, showed that both oils lacked activity against any of the bacteria. However, *Eucalyptus globulus* was more active against the yeast species, particularly *Candida albicans*.

The two oils extracted from woods, namely cedarwood and sandalwood, showed very low activity against all organisms tested.

Jasmine absolute and ylang ylang essential oil showed only very low activities against *S. pombe*.

METHOD OF TESTING I – DROP DIFFUSION

Consistency in agar thickness was achieved on all the plates. Then all organisms were grown to a consistent population density and a measured amount of culture was spread evenly onto the plates.

In order to reduce the variability due to sample size, 0.5 ml of the test oil was applied as a single drop to the centre of each plate.

For accurate comparisons it was important that the measuring of inhibition zones was within 30 minutes of the end of incubation in order to ensure that the organisms were in a consistent phase of growth when testing different oils. It has been previously shown that inhibition zones will vary depending on the time exposure.

The rate of diffusion of the essential oils on the agar plates was not measured. Antimicrobial agents generally need to contact the microorganisms in order to inhibit their growth. Using this technique an essential oil with low volatility, which is insoluble in the media, may falsely show no activity. The volatility of an essential oil will also influence its ability to contact microorganisms and inhibit their growth.

A study examining the activity of hyssop oil against the bacterium *Sarcina ureae* used the agar overlay technique and a technique where the activity of the vapour alone was tested. The oil inhibited *Sarcina ureae* completely using agar overlayed with a paper disc, whereas the oil vapour was not at all active.

One of the major concerns regarding assay techniques is that the drop diffusion technique is mostly used as the preliminary screening prior to the use of broth dilution techniques. It is possible using this strategy that among the oils rejected for further investigation there is an oil with high antimicrobial activity in dilution. Future work should involve looking at a larger range of oils using both techniques.

METHOD OF TESTING II – BROTH DILUTION

In order to get more detailed information, broth dilution assays were conducted on 13 of the essential oils showing most activity in the drop diffusion technique. The oils chosen were:

Cardamom (*Elettaria cardamomum*)
Cinnamon (*Cinnamomum zeylanicum*)
Clove (*Eugenia caryophyllata*)
Coriander (*Coriandrum sativum*)
Ho leaf (*Cinnamomum camphora*)
Lemongrass (*Cymbopogon citratus*)
Marjoram, Spanish (*Thymus mastichina*)
Palmarosa (*Cymbopogon martinii*)
Peppermint (*Piper nigrum*)
Rosemary *(Rosmarinus officinalis)*
Sage (*Salvia officinalis*)
Tea tree (*Melaleuca alternifolia*)
Thyme (*Thymus vulgaris*)

The essential oils were diluted into a range of concentrations using DMSO as a solubiliser. DMSO was chosen as the solubiliser after preliminary tests that showed that DMSO did not itself inhibit the growth of the microorganisms.

The range of concentrations used for testing antimicrobial activity was 10, 50, 100, 200, 300, 400 and 500 $\mu g\ ml^{-1}$. The general trend was for the antimicrobial activity of the oils to increase with increasing concentration and for this reason only the 500 μg ml^{-1} is shown.

% REDUCTION IN GROWTH CAUSED BY ESSENTIAL OILS AT 500 μG ML-1 IN BROTH DILUTION

	Bacteria			Yeasts			
	E. Coli	*S. aureus*	*P. aerugenosa*	*C. albicans*	*S. pombe*	*S. cerevisiae*	*T. utilus*
Cardamom	46	59	44	41	82	90	62
Cinnamon	67	70	85	72	96	59	100
Clove	74	83	75	61	94	99	95
Coriander	67	44	74	75	18	68	87
Ho Leaf	48	19	56	5	32	19	26
Lemongrass	67	86	71	42	0	96	81
Marjoram, Sp.	0	29	14	20	71	94	12
Palmarosa	42	47	63	71	100	100	100
Peppermint	57	42	66	71	100	100	100
Rosemary	36	1	54	8	87	88	2
Sage	25	17	62	17	0	8	50
Tea Tree	28	43	75	37	74	69	33
Thyme	75	95	77	100	100	100	100

Table 4. Figures refer to a minimum of 3 replicates

There was some variation in data from the drop diffusion assay compared with that from the broth dilution method. For example, using the drop diffusion assay rosemary and sage oils showed no activity against *P. aerugenosa*, but using the broth dilution assay, a 53.5 % and 61.5 % reduction in growth was observed respectively. The diameter of the inhibition zone in the drop diffusion test for cinnamon oil against *S. cerevisiae* and *T. utilus* was similar at 53 mm and 42.3 mm respectively, whereas in the broth dilution assay a 59 % and 100 % reduction in cell growth was recorded respectively. On drop diffusion assays, palmarosa oil showed no activity against *E. coli*, but in dilution techniques caused a reduction in growth of 42.2 %.

In summary, essential oils in dilution and those that come into physical contact with microorganisms were more effective in their antimicrobial activity than essential oils used as a single drop and reliant partly on vapour diffusion.

Chapter 3

Comparison of Components and Complete Oils

The argument about whether isolated constituents or the whole plant is better has raged in herbal medicine and aromatherapy for many years. The trend in modern science and by extension modern medicine has been to seek 'active constituents' and then extract them for use or synthesise them. Those involved in 'wholistic medicine' have argued that the whole plant is better; either because the many constituents present in a plant are thought to work synergistically together, or because the whole plant has some 'vital' energy that is not present in an isolate.

Research was undertaken to compare the antimicrobial activity of certain major components with their associated essential oils. In the past, certain components have been isolated for use as antimicrobials. For example, thymol found in thyme essential oil was in the past widely used as a hospital and clinic disinfectant.

The antimicrobial activities of pure thymol, 1-8 cineol, eugenol and linalool were also tested. The amount of these components in each oil was estimated. Concentrations equivalent to the amount found in 500 ug ml-1 of oil were compared with 500 ug ml-1 of oil to examine how much of the antimicrobial activity of the oils was attributable to a single component. Triplicate experiments were conducted and the antimicrobial activity of the component and the oil compared. Table 4 shows the percentage reduction in growth caused by the pure compounds and the oils at a concentration of 500 mg ml-1.

% REDUCTION IN GROWTH CAUSED BY ESSENTIAL OILS AT 500MCG ML(-1) AND THEIR MAJOR COMPONENTS

	Bacteria			Yeasts			
	E. Coli	*S. aureus*	*P. aerugenosa*	*C. albicans*	*S. pombe*	*S. cerevisiae*	*T. utilus*
Clove oil	55	54	28	20	47	50	51
Eugenol	40	21	22	19	80	35	51
Cinnamon oil	39	37	17	30	49	46	56
Eugenol	25	1	0	5	37	15	45
Thyme oil	45	58	0	73	72	77	74
Thymol	20	2	0	7	40	38	17
Cardamom oil	27	12	16	10	92	91	48
1-8 Cineole	7	3	10	1	0	0	0
Coriander	12	10	0	7	86	92	26
Linalool	10	0	0	0	17	6	18

Antimicrobial activity of clove oil was compared with eugenol, present in the clove oil at above 68%. No significant difference at the 95% confidence level existed between the activity of clove oil and eugenol against *C. albicans, S. cerevisiae, T. utilus* and *P. aerugenosa* suggesting the antimicrobial activity of clove oil against these organisms was solely due to the antimicrobial activity of eugenol. Against *E. coli* and *S. aureus* clove oil showed higher antimicrobial activity and against *S. pombe* eugenol's antimicrobial activity was significantly higher than that of clove oil.

The antimicrobial activity of thyme oil was compared with thymol, a major component forming 33% of the oil. Thyme oil showed significantly higher activity against all organisms suggesting that components other than thymol are contributing to the antimicrobial activity of thyme oil. Other components that are found in thyme oil and that are known to have activity include carvacrol and terpineol.

The antimicrobial activity of cardamom was compared with 1-8 cineole, present in cardamom at 23%. Cardamom showed significantly higher activity against *S. cerevisiae, T. utilus* and *S. pombe* as 1-8 cineole had no inhibitory effects on the growth of these organisms. No significant differences existed between cardamom and 1-8 cineole against *C. albicans, E. coli, S. aureus* and *P. aerugenosa.*

The antimicrobial activity of coriander was compared with linalool which is present in coriander at 63.5 %. Significant differences in activity were only found with *S. cerevisiae* and *S. pombe.* For all other organisms no significant difference existed between the activity of coriander oil and linalool.

The antimicrobial activity of cinnamom oil was compared with eugenol which is present in cinnamon oil at 50 %. Cinnamon oil showed significantly higher antimicrobial activity against *C. albicans, S. cerevisiae, T. utilus, S. pombe* and *S. aureus* suggesting other components were contributing to its antimicrobial activity. Against *E. coli* and *P. aerugenosa* no significant difference existed between cinnamon oil and eugenol.

SUMMARY

Generally speaking, the complete essential oil had a greater antimicrobial effect against a wider variety of microorganisms than the isolated constituents.

The other point that should be made is that this is an in vitro experiment and directly relevant to using essential oils as disinfectants. Where essential oils are used on living organisms there is another effect that must be taken into account; that of immune system enhancement. This is a further argument for using essential oils as a whole rather than isolating constituents.

RECIPES

The following recipes are based on essential oils selected for their appropriateness in treating the specific micro-organisms associated with particular conditions.

ORAL CARE

BLEEDING GUM GEL

0.5g	pectin
20ml	vegetable glycerine
40ml	chamomile infusion
5 drops	myrrh tincture
5 drops	raspberry tincture
1 drop	clove oil
1 drop	cinnamon oil

Method

1. Make up chamomile infusion using a chamomile tea bag or a heaped teaspoon of herb, leave to stand for 10 minutes and strain before using.
2. Add the pectin to the chamomile infusion and heat gently until all the pectin has dissolved.
3. Add in the glycerine and mix well
4. Add in the tinctures and essential oils.
5. Store in the fridge to avoid product spoilage.

BREATH FRESHENING MOUTH RINSE

60ml	glycerine
38ml	water
2 drops	peppermint oil
1 drop	thyme oil
2 drops	lavender oil
1 drop	cinnamon oil
4 drops	spearmint oil

Method
1. Add essential oils to the glycerine and mix well.
2. While continuously stirring slowly add in the water.
3. Store in a clean glass jar and shake well before use.

TOOTHPASTE

25g	bicarbonate of soda
3ml	water
1 drop	spearmint oil
1 drop	clove oil
2 drops	lemon oil

Method
1. Weigh out bicarbonate of soda
2. Add enough water to make a smooth paste
3. Add in essential oils
4. Store in an appropriate container eg small jar

NB Calcium carbonate or clay can be used to replace the bicarbonate if preferred.

SKIN CARE

When using products designed to help with acne it is important to remember that acne is caused by bacteria and thus ensure that the hands and face are clean prior to applying these products to the skin. The most appropriate way to apply these products is on the end of a cotton bud or using cotton wool rather than your fingers. Always wash skin well using one of the cleansing formulas given prior to applying the acne treatments.

ACNE TREATMENT FOR DRY SKIN

A simple formula to make. Apply using a cotton bud after cleansing.

5 drops	palmarosa oil
2 drops	tea tree oil
1 drop	cajeput oil
2 drops	juniper oil
3 drops	jasmine absolute
25ml	carrot oil
25ml	calendula macerated oil

Method

1. Mix together the essential oils
2. In a seperate bowl mix together the base oils
3. Slowly add the essential oils to the base oils with mixing
4. Store in a glass container

ACNE CREAM FOR DRY SKIN

A more complex formula to make. Apply where required after cleansing.

8g	self emulsifying wax
5ml	jojoba oil
5ml	wheatgerm oil
70ml	infusion of yarrow and thyme
10ml	rosewater
1 drop	lavender oil
1 drop	juniper oil

2 drop	palmarosa oil
3 drops	jasmine absolute
1 drop	tea tree oil

Method
1. Weigh out self emulsifying wax and jojoba and calendula oil into a heat proof bowl (OIL PHASE).
2. Weigh out the infusion and rosewater into a separate heat proof bowl (WATER PHASE).
3. Heat both the oil phase and the water phase to 70°C
4. Slowly add the oil phase to the water phase with constant mixing
5. A white smooth cream should result
6. Allow the cream to cool to room temperature
7. Add in essential oils with mixing
8. NOTE this product should be kept in the fridge to prevent spoilage

ACNE TREATMENT FOR ALL SKIN TYPES

A simple formula. Apply locally.

40g	shea nut butter
40g	lanolin
10ml	carrot oil
10 drops	jasmine absolute
10 drops	palmarosa oil
5 drops	tea tree oil

Method
1. Melt the sheanut butter and the lanolin over hot water
2. Add in the carrot oil and mix well
3. Add in the essential oils with constant mixing until cooled
4. Pour into glass jars

ACNE TREATMENT FOR OILY SKIN

Apply using cotton wool after cleansing.

2 drops	palmarosa oil
2 drops	tea tree oil
1 drop	clove oil
2 drops	lavender oil
1 drop	marjoram oil
10 drops	propolis tincture
2ml	glycerine
100ml	witchazel

Method

1. Add the essential oils to the glycerine with mixing
2. Add propolis and continue to mix
3. Slowly add the glycerine mixture to the witchazel with constant mixing
4. Pour into an appropriate container.
5. NOTE: This product may require vigourous shaking prior to each use to redisperse the essential oils

ACNE GEL FOR ALL SKIN TYPES

Apply locally where required.

0.5 g	agar agar
20ml	infusion of rosemary
1 teaspoon	lemon juice
10ml	witchazel
70ml	water
1 drop	palmarosa oil
1 drop	cajuput oil
3 drops	lavender oil

Method

1. Make rosemary infusion using 1 teaspoon of herb to half a cup of boiling water, leave to stand for 10 minutes and strain.
2. Mix together rosemary infusion, lemon juice, witchazel and water.
3. Add agar agar and heat with constant mixing until all the agar has dissolved.

4. Remove from the heat and allow to cool slowly.
5. When the mixture is at room temperature mix in essential oils with vigorous stirring.
6. Store in a jar in the refrigerator.

WASH OFF CLEANSER FOR OILY SKIN

A soap based cleanser for oily or problem skin. Apply to damp skin and rinse off with tepid water.

5g	grated soap
10ml	glycerine
10ml	rosewater
40ml	infusion of peppermint
40ml	spring water
10 drops	lemon oil
5 drops	ho leaf oil
2 drops	lavender oil

Method

1. Add rosewater, spring water and peppermint infusion together.
2. Add grated soap and mix with gentle heating until the soap has dissolved.
3. Allow to cool to room temperature.
4. Add essential oils to the glycerine and then slowly add to the cooled soap mixture with constant mixing.
5. Store in a glass container.
6. Note: this product will need to be shaken before each use to ensure the essential oils are well dissolved.

WASH OFF CLEANSER FOR DRY SKIN

Apply to the skin using fingertips or cotton wool and rinse off with tepid water.

10g	self emulsifying wax
5ml	avocado oil
5ml	calendula macerated oil
3g	grated beeswax
60ml	calendula infusion
10ml	glycerine
2 drops	propolis tincture
2 drops	cajuput oil
2 drops	juniper oil
2 drops	lavender oil

Method

1. Measure out self emulsifying wax and avocado and calendula oil into a heat proof bowl (OIL PHASE)
2. Measure out the infusion and glycerine into another heat proof bowl (WATER PHASE)
3. Heat both the oil phase and the water phase to 70°C
4. Slowly add the oil phase to the water phase with constant mixing
5. A white smooth cream should result
6. Allow the cream to cool to room temperature
7. Add in essential oils with mixing
8. NOTE this product should be kept in the fridge to prevent spoilage

CLEANSING FACE SCRUB

An excellent way to exfoliate and cleanse the skin. Suitable for all skin types. To use place a small amount of scrub in the palm of the hand, mix with a little water and apply to the skin using small circular movements. Rinse off with tepid water.

10g	clay eg bentonite, kaolin, green clay
10g	ground rice
2ml	clear honey
Juice	1 lemon
2g	ground rosemary herb

Spring water to create a paste	
3 drops	orange oil
3 drops	lemon oil
3 drops	peppermint oil

Method
1. Combine all dry ingredients and mix well.
2. Add in honey and lemon juice.
3. Add enough spring water to make a paste
4. Add in essential oils and mix well.
5. NB this mixture will harden with time and is best prepared just before use.

CLEANSING FACE MASK

A purifying mask for normal or oily skin. Apply to the skin, leave on for 10-15 minutes and rinse off with tepid water.

0.5g	carrageenan (or agar or similar thickener)
45ml	lavender flower water
2ml	clear honey
5ml	sage tincture
35g	kaolin or other clay
5 drops	palmarosa oil
1 drop	coriander oil
2 drops	thyme oil

Method
1. Make up infusion.
2. Add carrageenan to the infusion and dissolve well.
3. Add honey and sage tincture and mix well.
4. With constant stirring add enough kaolin until a thick paste forms.
5. Add in essential oils and mix well.
6. Keep refrigerated.

SCAR TREATMENT OIL

A regenerative oil blend for helping to break down scar tissue. It may also be used as an effective anti-wrinkle blend. Massage in gently to required areas.

10ml	rosehip oil or calendula macerated oil
30ml	organic olive oil
5 drops	neroli oil
5 drops	rose oil

Method

1. Measure out rosehip/calendula oil and olive oil
2. Add in essential oils and mix well
3. Apply as required

ANTIBACTERIAL SKIN TONER

This antiseptic skin toner may be applied after cleansing by using cotton wool, or it works really well if you use it from an atomiser.

50ml	witch hazel
30ml	glycerine
30ml	spring water
3 drops	juniper oil
2 drops	lemon oil
4 drops	orange oil
5 drops	palmarosa oil

Method

1. Measure out essential oils
2. Measure out glycerine
3. With constant mixing add essential oils to the glycerine
4. Mix together the infusion, witch hazel and spring water
5. Add glycerine and essential oil mixture to the infusion, witch hazel and spring water mixture.
6. Add to bottle and shake well before each use

REGENERATIVE MOISTURISER FOR DRY SKIN

8g	self emulsifying wax
8ml	apricot kernel oil
5ml	wheatgerm oil
2g	grated beeswax
1 Vitamin E oil capsule broken open and emptied into the wheatgerm oil	
50ml	spring water
5ml	clear honey
10ml	rosewater
1 drop	patchouli oil
2 drops	geranium oil
1 drop	frankincense oil

Method

1. Measure out self emulsifying wax, beeswax, apricot and wheatgerm oil into a heat proof bowl (OIL PHASE)
2. Measure out the spring water, honey and rosewater into another heat proof bowl (WATER PHASE)
3. Heat both the oil phase and the water phase to 70°C
4. Slowly add the oil phase to the water phase with constant mixing
5. A white smooth cream should result
6. Allow the cream to cool to room temperature
7. Add in essential oils with mixing
8. NOTE this product should be kept in the fridge to prevent spoilage

ANTIBACTERIAL FACE WIPES

Handy 'wet-wipes' that can be used to cleanse or refresh the skin.

10 cotton wool face pads (if these are unavailable cotton wool balls will suffice)	
3 drops	sage oil
5 drops	lavender oil
4 drops	juniper oil
1 drop	tea tree oil
10ml	glycerine
30ml	aloe vera juice

Method
1. Place face pads in a container in which they will fit snuggly
2. Mix essential oils into the glycerine
3. Slowly add in aloe vera juice with constant stirring
4. Pour mixture over the cotton face pads, allow to soak in, and seal for use

COLD SORE/ LIP OIL

An anti-viral blend to dab on to cold sores, or apply to the lips as a conditioning oil.

10ml	calendula macerated oil
5 drops	tea tree oil
5 drops	orange oil
5 drops	lemon
2 drops	thyme linanol oil

Method
1. Measure out calendula oil
2. Add in essential oils and mix well

ANTIBACTERIAL WIPES FOR CHILDREN

Soothing and antiseptic tissues suitable for children.

30 tissues	
10ml	calendula tincture
5 drops	lavender oil
2 drops	rose absolute
5 drops	Roman chamomile oil
40ml	glycerine

Method
1. Place tissues into a container in which they will fit snuggly
2. Mix essential oils into the glycerine
3. Slowly add in the calendula tincture
4. Pour mixture over the tissues and seal for use

HAIR CARE

DANDRUFF SHAMPOO

100ml	bottle of basic shampoo
10 drops	rosemary oil
5 drops	cedarwood oil

Method
1. Add essential oils to the shampoo base with constant mixing
2. Shampoo hair as normally

ANTI-DANDRUFF TREATMENT OIL

5 drops	lavender oil
10 drops	cedarwood oil
2 drops	lemon oil
1 drop	thyme oil
100ml	jojoba oil

Method
1. Measure out jojoba oil
2. Add in essential oils and mix well
3. Apply a small amount to hair, massage into scalp and comb through well. Leave on for at least 2 hours before washing out.

HAIR STYLING WAX

50g	lanolin
10g	sheanut butter
5 drops	cedarwood oil
2 drops	ylang ylang oil

Method
1. Weigh out lanolin and sheanut butter and melt over boiling water.
2. Add in essential oils and mix well until solidified.
3. Place in a jar for regular use.

DEODORISING HAIR SPRAY

Excellent for freshening hair which has been in a smoky pub.

50ml	aloe vera juice
10ml	glycerine
1 drop of	lavender oil
1 drop	jasmine absolute
3 drops	clary sage oil

Method
1. Add essential oils to the glycerine and mix very well.
2. Slowly add in the aloe vera juice with constant mixing
3. Place in atomised container and shake well before use.

ANTI-DANDRUFF CONDITIONING RINSE

Apply to the hair after shampooing. Massage into the scalp and comb through the hair, leave on for 10 minutes, rinse off.

8g	self emulsifying wax
2ml	wheatgerm oil
5ml	calendula macerated or olive oil
1g	grated beeswax
90ml	spring water
5ml	honey
1 drop	lemon oil
2	drops orange oil
1	drop thyme oil

Method
1. Measure out self emulsifying wax, beeswax and base oils into a heat proof bowl (OIL PHASE)
2. Weigh out the spring water and honey into another heat proof bowl (WATER PHASE)
3. Heat both the oil phase and the water phase to 70 degrees C
4. Slowly add oil phase to water phase with constant mixing
5. A white smooth cream should result
6. Allow the cream to cool to room temperature
7. Add in essential oils with mixing
8. NOTE this product should be kept in the fridge to prevent spoilage

BODY CARE

ANTI-FUNGAL FOOT SCRUB

50ml	infusion of thyme herb
0.5 g	pectin
40g	kaolin
1 drop	lemon oil
5 drops	ho leaf oil
3 drops	palmarosa oil
4 drops	ginger oil
6 drops	peppermint oil

Method

1. Make up the infusion by using two teaspoonfuls of thyme, add boiling water, stand for 10 minutes and strain
2. Add in pectin and stir with gentle heating until all has dissolved
3. Add in kaolin
5. Add essential oils and mix well
6. Store in glass jar in the refrigerator

DEODORANT (MASCULINE FRAGRANCE)

60ml	alcohol (either ethanol or vodka)
40ml	glycerine
3 drops	clove oil
2 drops	cinnamon oil
1 drop	tea tree oil
8 drops	lemongrass oil

Method

1. Add essential oils to alcohol and mix well
2. Slowly add in glycerine and continue to mix well
3. Add to glass bottle with atomiser spray and shake well before each use

DEODORANT (FEMININE FRAGRANCE)

60ml	alcohol (ethanol or vodka)
40ml	glycerine
5 drops	rose absolute
2 drops	jasmine absolute
4 drops	ho leaf oil
2 drops	coriander oil

Method
1. Add essential oils to alcohol and mix well
2. Slowly add in glycerine and continue to mix well
3. Add to glass bottle with atomiser spray and shake well before each use

CANDIDA RINSE

An anti-fungal lotion. Make up fresh each day and apply with cotton wool.

20ml	infusion of thyme herb
3ml	glycerine
10ml	golden seal tincture
1 drop	sage oil
3 drops	palmarosa oil

Method
1. Make up thyme infusion using a heaped teaspoon of thyme herb, add boiling water, strain and cool.
2. In a separate bowl add essential oils to the glycerine and mix well
3. Slowly add in thyme infusion and mix well

ANTI-FUNGAL CREAM

A soothing anti-fungal cream to apply as required. Suitable for thrush, ringworm, athlete's foot and other fungal infections.

40g	unfragranced zinc and castor oil baby barrier cream, or other ointment base.
10 drops	palmarosa oil
1 drop	tea tree oil
3 drops	lavender oil

Method

1. Add essential oils to the baby barrier and mix well

CHEST RUB

A blend of antiseptic and decongestant oils to apply to the chest or add to hot water and inhale the vapours.

10g	grated beeswax
80ml	calendula macerated oil
3 drops	cypress oil
5 drops	eucalyptus oil
4 drops	rosemary oil

Method

1. Measure out beeswax and calendula oil
2. Melt over a gentle heat
3. Add in essential oils and allow to cool slowly with continuous mixing
4. Pour into a jar ready for use

ANTIBACTERIAL SOAP

600g	coconut oil
200g	cocoa butter
450ml	thyme infusion
150g	sodium hydroxide
5ml	lemongrass oil
5ml	palmarosa oil
1ml	clove leaf oil
2ml	tea tree oil

Method

1. Place coconut oil and cocoa butter into a stainless steel pot over a low heat.
2. Pour infusion into a plastic bowl
3. Wearing gloves and eye protection add the sodium hydroxide to the water and stir until dissolved
4. When coconut oil and cocoa butter have melted, remove from heat
5. Place a thermometer in the oils and one in the caustic solution
6. When both temperatures reach about 55° C pour the caustic solution into the oil with constant mixing
7. Stir occasionally until the soap begins to thicken
8. Add in essential oils
9. Pour into a mould and cover with a towel
10. Leave to set for 24 hours or until the soap becomes solid
11. Remove from mould and cut into bars.
12. Allow to 'cure' for 4 weeks before use

Appendix I

REFERENCES TO CHAPTER 1

Bacillus cereus

Author: Meena and Sethi
Title: Antimicrobial Activity of Essential Oils from Spices
Journal: Journal of Food Science and Technology, 1994, Volume 31, No. 1, 68-70.

Pseudomonas aerugenosa

Author: Panizzi, L., Famini, G., Gioni, P.L. and Morelli, I.
Title: Composition and antimicrobial Properties of Essential Oils of Four Mediterranean Lamiaceae
Journal: Journal of Ethnopharmacy, 1993, Volume 39, 167-170.

Escherichia coli

Author: Smith Palmer, A., Stewart, J., Fyfe, L.
Title: Antimicrobial Properties of Plant Essential Oils and Essences Against Five Food-borne Pathogens
Journal: Letters in Applied Microbiology, 1998, Volume 26, No. 2, 118-122.

Salmonella enterititis

Author: Hammer, K.A., Carson, C.F., Riley, T.V.
Title: Antimicrobial Activity of Essential Oils and Other Plant Extracts
Journal: Journal of Applied Microbiology, 1999, Volume 86, No. 6, 985-990.

Propionibacteria

Author: Raman, A., Weir, U., Bloomfield, S.F.
Title: Antimicrobial Effects of Tea Tree Oil and its Major Components on Staph. aureus, Staph. epidermas and Propionbacterium Acnes

Leptotrichia buccalis

Author: Shaphiro, S., Meier, A., Guggenheim, B.
Title: The Antimicrobial Activity of Essential Oils and Essential Oil Components Towards Oral Bacteria
Journal: Oral Microbiology and Immunology, 1994, Volume 9 (4), 202-208.

Streptococcus mutans

Author: Branchmays, Z.G., Hao, J., Laffoon, J., and Wu Yuan, C.D.
Title: Antimicrobial Activity of Plant Essential Oils Against Oral Pathogens
Journal: Journal of Dental Research, 73, (IADR Abstracts).

Pityrosporum ovale

Author: Nenoff, P., Haustein, U.F., Brandt, W.
Title: Antifungal Activity of the Essential Oil of Melaleuca alternifolia (Tea Tree) Against Pathogenic Fungi in vitro
Journal: Skin Pharmacology, 1996, 9 (6), 388-394.

Trichophyton mentagophytes,

Trichophyton violaceam
Author: Kishore, N., Mishra, A.K. and Chansouria, J.P.N.
Title: Fungitoxicity of Essential Oils Against Dermatophytes
Journal: Mycoses, 1993, (36), 211-215.

Candida albicans

Author: Suresh, B., Sriram, S., Dhanaraj, S.A., Elango, K., Chinnaswamy, K.
Journal: Journal of Ethnopharmacology, 1997, June, 55 (2), 151-159.

Bibliography

Al Saadawi, I.S., Arif, M.B., Al Rubeaa, A.J., (1985), Allelopathic effects of Citrus aurantium L, 2, Isolation, Characterisation, and Biological Activities of Phytotoxins, Journal of Chemical Ecology, 11, 1527-1534.

Bard, M., Albrecht, M.R., Gupta, N., Guynn, C.J., and Stillwell, W., (1988) Geraniol interferes with membrane functions in strains of Candida and Saccharomyces, Lipids, 23, 6, 534-538.

Bean, N.H., Griffin, P.M., Goulding, J.S., and Ivey, C.B., (1990), Foodborne Disease Outbreaks, 5 year summary, 1983-1987, Journal of Food Protection, 53, 711-728.

Bonner, A., (1991), The Biogenesis of Natural Compounds, ed Bernfield, P., p. 241, Pergamon Press.

Carson, C.F., and Riley, T.V., (1995). Antimicrobial Activity of the Major Components of the Essential Oil of Melaleuca alternifolia, Journal of Applied Bacteriology, 78, 264-269.

Cruz, T., Cabo, M., Castillo, M.J., and Jumenez, J., (1993). Chemical Composition and Antimicrobial Activity of the Essential Oils of Different Samples of Thymus baeticus Boiss, Phytotherapy Research , 7, 92-94.

Curtis, C.F., Lines, J.D., Ijumba, J., Callaghan, A., Hill, N., and Karimzad, M.A., (1987), The Relative Efficiency of Repellants Against Mosquito Vectors of Disease, Med. Veter. Entomol., 1, 109-119.

Cutler, H.G., (1995) Natural Product Flavour Compounds as Potential Antimicrobials, Insecticides and Medicinals. Agra-food Industry Hi Tech, 6, 4, 19-23.

Cuvelier, M.E., Berset, C., and Richard, H., (1994). Antioxidant Constituents in Sage (Salvia officinalis), Journal of Agricultural and Food Chemistry, 42, 665-669.

Dixshit, A., Singh, A.K., Dixit, S.A., (1992). Effect of pH on Fungistatic Activity of Some Essential Oils, Bokin Bobai, 10,1, 9-10.

Duke, S.O., (1987). Terpenoids from the Genus Artemisia as Potential Pesticides. Abs. Papers Am. Chem. Soc. 194, 104.

Dwivedi, S.K., and Dubey, N.K., (1993), Potential Use of the Essential Oil of Trachyspermum ammi Against Seed-borne Fungi of Guar (Cyamopsis tetragonoloba L. (Taub.)). Mycopathologia, 121, 101-104.

Ghfit, B., Fonvielle, J.L., Koulali, Y., Ecalle, R., and Dargent, R., (1994). Effect of Essential Oil of Hyssopus officinalis on Lipid Composition of Aspergillus fumigatus, Mycopathologia, 126, (3), 163-167.

Gould, M.N., (1995), Prevention and Therapy of Mammary Cancer by Monoterpenes. Journal of Cellular Biochemistry, 522, 139-144.

Grgesania, D., Mandic, M.L., Kanisa, L., Klapec, T., Bockinac, D., (1995), Chemical Composition of Different Parts of Matricaria chamomilla, Prehrambeno Tehnoloska I Biotehnoloska Revija 33, 2-3, 111-113.

Janseen, A.M., Scheffer, J.J.C., and Svendsen, A.B., (1987). Antimicrobial Activity of Essential Oils: A 1976-1986 Literature Review Aspects of Test Methods, Planta Medica, 53, 395-398.

Jay, J.M., and Rivers, G.M. (1984), Antimicrobial Activity of Some Food Flavouring Compounds, Journal of Food Safety, 6, 129-139.

Kim, J.M., Marshall, M.R., and Wei, C., (1995), Antibacterial Activity of Some Essential Oil Components Against 5 Foodborne Pathogens, J. Agric. Food. Chem., 45, 2839-2845.

Lawrence, B.M., (1978), Essential Oils, Allured Publishing, USA.

Lima, E.D., Gomertz, O.F., Paulo, M.D., Giesrecht, A.M., (1992). In vitro Antifungal Activity of Essential Oils Against Clinical Isolates of Dermatophytes, Revista de Microbiolgia, 23, (4), 235-238.

Martindale, W. (1910) The Chemistry and Manufacture of Cosmetics, Allured Publishers, USA., Vol. 3 pp 85-109.

Moore, E., (1997), Killer Bacteria, Guardian, p.1, 14 January 1997.

Morris, J.A., Khettry, A., and Seitz, E.W., (1979), Antimicrobial Activity of Aroma Chemicals and Essential Oils, Journal of the American Oil Chemists Society, 56, 595-603.

Pandey, V.N., and Dubey, N.K., (1994) Antifungal Potential of Leaves and Essential Oils from Higher Plants Against Soil Phytopathogens, Soil Biology and Biochemistry, 26, (10), 1,417-1421.

Panizzi, L., Flamini, G., Gioni, P.L., and Morelli, I., (1993) Composition and Antimicrobial Properties of Essential Oils of Four Mediterranean Lamiaceae, Journal of Ethnopharmacology, 39, 167-170.

Patkar, K.L., Usha, C.M., Shetty, H.S., Paster, N., and Lacey, J., (1993), Effect of Spice Essential Oil on Growth and Aflatoxin B1 Production by Aspergillus flavus, Letters in Applied Microbiology, 17, (2), 49-51.

Pellecuer, J., Jacob, M., de Buochberg, S., Dusart, G., Atlisto, M., Barthez, M., Gourgas, L., Pascal, B., and Tomei, B., (1980). Essais d'utilitisation d'huiles essentielles de plantes aromatiques mediterraneennes en odontologie conservatrice, Plant Med. Phytotherapie, 14, 83-98.

Price, S., and Price, L., (1993), Therapeutic Aspects of Essential Oils, Society of Cosmetic Scientists and British Society of Perfumers Symposium on Fragrance - more than just a pleasant smell. Paper 11.

Rose, A.H., and Veazey, F.J., (1988) Yeast a Practical Approach, 1st ed., Edited by Campbell, I., and Duffus, J.H., IRL Press, Oxford, Washington DC, pp 225-275.

Rose, J.E., and Behm, F.M., (1994) Inhalation of Vapour from Black Pepper Extract Reduces Smoking Withdrawal Symptoms, Drug and Alcohol Dependance, 34, 225-229.

Sarac, A. and Tunc, I., (1995). Toxicity of Essential Oil Vapour to Stored Product Insects, Journal of Plant Disease and Protection, 102, (1), 69-74.

Schreck, C.E., and Leonhardt, B.A., (1991), Efficacy Assessment of Quiwenling, a Mosquito Repellent from China, J. American Mosquito Control Assoc., 7, (3), 433-436.

Senatore, F., (1996). Influence of Harvesting Time on Yield and Composition of a Thyme (Thymus pulegiodes L.) Growing Wild in Campania (Southern Italy). Journal of Agricultural Food Chemistry 44, 1327-1332.

Simeon de Buochberg, M., Allegrini, J., Bessiere, M., Attisto, J., Passet, M., and Granger, R., (1976). Prorietes Microbiologiques des Huiles Essentielles de Chimiotypes de Thymus vulgaris Linnaeus, Riv. Ital. EPPOS, 58, 527-536.

Sivropoulou, A., Papanikolaou, E., Nikolaou, C., Kokkini, S., Lanaras, T., and Arsenakis, M., (1996). Antimicrobial and Cytotoxic Activities of Origanum Essential Oils, J. Agric. Food Chem., 44, 1202-1205.

Steinmetz, M.D., Moulin-Traffort, J., and Regli, P., (1988), Transmission and Scanning Electronmicroscopy Study of the Action of Sage and Rosemary Essential Oils and Eucalyptol on Candida albicans, Mycoses, 31,1, 40-51.

Subba, M.S., Soumithri, T.C., and Suryanarayana, R., (1967), Antimicrobial Action of Citrus Oils., J. Food Science, 32, 225-227.

Suresh, P., Ingle, V.K., Vijajlakshimi, V., (1992) Antimicrobial Activity of Eugenol in Comparison with Other Antibiotics, J. Food Sci. Technol. 29, 254-256.

Tantaoui-Elarki, A., and Errifi, A., (1994). Antifungal Activity of Essential Oils When Associated with Sodium Chloride or Fatty Acids, Grasas. Y Aceities, 45, (6), 363-369.

Trigg, J.K. and Hill, N., (1996) Laboratory Evaluation of a Eucalyptus Based Repellent Against Four Biting Arthropods, Phytotherapy Research, 10, 313-316.

Valentin, A., Pelissier, Y., Benoit, F., Marion, C., Kone, D., Mallie, M., Bastide, J.M., Bissiere, J.M., (1995). Composition and Antimalarial Activity of in vitro of Volatile Components of Lippia multiflora, Phytochemistry, 40, (5), 1439-1442.

Viollon, C., and Chaumont, J.P., (1994). Antifungal Properties of Essential Oils and Their Main Components upon Crytococcus neoformans, Mycopathologia, 128, 151-153.

Williams, D.G., (1996), The Chemistry of Essential Oils, Micelle Press.

Witte, L., (1986) Gas chromatography/Mass spectrometry - Modern Methods of Plant Analysis, ed. Linskens, H.F., and Jackson, J.F., Springer Verlag. New York, Tokyo, pp 134-145

Yousef, R., and Tawil, G., (1980) Antimicrobial activity of Volatile Oils. Pharmazie, 35, 698-701.

USEFUL CONTACTS

Aromatherapy Organisations Council
Provides a national register of qualified aromatherapists and addresses of training establishments.
The Secretary AOC
PO Box 19824
London SE25 6WF
Tel: 020 8251 7912
www.aoc.uk.net

Aromatherapy Trade Council
A trade organisation of essential oil suppliers that will provide a list of reputable suppliers and further information.
The Secretary ATC
PO Box 387
Ipswich IP2 9AN
Tel: 01473 603630
www.a-t-c.org.uk

SUPPLIERS

The quality of an essential oil used for therapeutic purposes is all important. You should establish the botanical name and country of origin of any oil purchased and buy only from reputable suppliers. The ATC (see previous page) supply a list of suppliers who conform to their criteria.

Neal's Yard Remedies supplies a range of high quality essential oils as used for the research in this book. They also supply a range of ingredients for making natural hair and skin care products like those used in the Recipes section.
Their products can be obtained in many parts of the world. Contact the UK Customer Services or website for details of your nearest outlet.

Neal's Yard Remedies
15 Neal's Yard
Covent Garden
London WC2H 9DP

Customer Services
020 7627 1949
email: cservices@nealsyardremedies.com

Mail Order
0161 831 7875
www.nealsyardremedies.com